HEARING WELLNESS

Ultimate Guide in Exploring Causes, Prevention, and Solutions to Hearing Health in the 21st Century

JENNIE BOSS

HEARING WELLNESS

By Jennie Boss MD

February 2024

© Mind Heal Publishing

All Rights Reserved

CONTENTS

INTRODUCTION

In the rich symphony of human existence, sound serves as the vibrant thread that weaves together our experiences, emotions, and connections with the world. From the gentle rustle of leaves in a summer breeze to the stirring crescendo of a concerto, our ability to perceive sound shapes our perceptions, enriches our lives, and forges bonds that transcend language and culture.

Yet, amidst the hustle and bustle of modern life, the intricate mechanisms of our auditory system often operate silently, unnoticed until the harmony of sound begins to falter. *Hearing Wellness* embarks on a profound exploration into the intricate realm of auditory health, offering a compendium of insights, guidance, and strategies to safeguard one of our most precious senses.

As we journey through the pages of this book, we venture into the labyrinthine landscape of hearing wellness, navigating through the myriad factors that influence its delicate balance. Our passage begins with an intimate exploration of the anatomy of hearing, unraveling the intricate interplay of nerves, cochlea, and auditory pathways that transform vibrations into the symphony of sensation.

From there, we embark on a voyage through the depths of understanding hearing loss, peeling back the layers of complexity to reveal the diverse array of factors – from genetic predispositions to environmental stressors—that can undermine our auditory acuity.

Chapter by chapter, we illuminate the shadows that obscure our understanding of hearing wellness, shedding light on the insidious impact of noise pollution, the silent menace of occupational hazards, and the inexorable march of age-related hearing loss. We probe into the web of genetics, exploring the complex interplay of hereditary factors that can shape our susceptibility to auditory challenges. With each revelation, we arm ourselves with knowledge, forging a bulwark of understanding against the tide of preventable hearing loss.

However, our journey does not end with mere illumination; it extends into the realm of action and advocacy, offering a roadmap for the preservation and enhancement of auditory health. From lifestyle choices that nurture the delicate mechanisms of the inner ear to the transformative potential of emerging technologies in hearing aids and assistive devices, we equip ourselves with the tools necessary to navigate the cacophony of modern existence with grace and resilience.

Yet, as we crisscross the landscape of Hearing Wellness, we are mindful of the profound social and psychological implications of hearing loss. From the isolation and stigma that can accompany auditory impairment to the ripple effects that reverberate through communities and families, we confront the human dimension of hearing health with empathy and compassion.

In the culmination of our journey, we embrace the imperative of advocacy and accessibility, championing the cause of equal hearing opportunities for all. Through education, outreach, and policy initiatives, we strive to dismantle the barriers that impede access to auditory health resources, ensuring that every voice is heard, every whisper cherished, and every melody resonates with clarity.

Join us on the Hearing Wellness cruise - a testament to the power of knowledge, compassion, and collective action in safeguarding one of humanity's most precious senses. Together, we embark on a voyage of discovery, empowerment, and transformation – a journey where the symphony of sound meets the harmony of health, and where every ear is attuned to the melody of life.

CHAPTER 1

THE ANATOMY OF HEARING

SECTION 1.1

THE WONDERS OF THE AUDITORY SYSTEM

The human auditory system is a marvel of precision and complexity, comprising a delicate network of structures that work in harmony to translate sound waves into meaningful sensory information. At the heart of this intricate mechanism lies the cochlea, a spiral-shaped organ nestled within the inner ear. Named after the Greek word for "snail shell," the cochlea is lined with thousands of specialized hair cells that detect vibrations and convert them into electrical signals. These signals are then relayed to the brain via the auditory nerve, where they are interpreted as the rich tapestry of sounds that shape our world.

Historically, the study of auditory anatomy dates back centuries, with pioneering figures such as Leonardo da Vinci and Andreas Vesalius laying the groundwork for our understanding of the inner workings of the ear. Through meticulous observation and dissection, these early anatomists unearthed the intricate structures that underpin our auditory perception, paving the way for modern research into hearing health.

SECTION 1.2

FROM SOUND WAVES TO SENSATION

The journey of sound through the auditory system is a symphony of precision and coordination, guided by a series of specialized structures and neural pathways. It begins with the external ear, where sound waves are collected and funneled through the ear canal to the eardrum. As the eardrum vibrates in response to sound, it sets into motion a chain of events that culminate in the activation of hair cells within the cochlea.

The cochlea itself is divided into three fluid-filled chambers, each responsive to different frequencies of sound. As sound waves travel through the cochlear fluid, they stimulate specific regions of the cochlear membrane, causing the hair cells to bend and generate electrical signals. These signals are then transmitted to the brainstem, where they are sorted, processed, and ultimately perceived as the diverse array of sounds that comprise our auditory landscape.

Throughout history, the study of auditory physiology has been marked by landmark discoveries and breakthroughs that have reshaped our understanding of hearing. From the pioneering experiments of Hermann von Helmholtz in the 19th century to the groundbreaking research of Georg von Békésy, whose work on cochlear mechanics earned him the Nobel Prize in Physiology or Medicine in 1961, our knowledge of the auditory system has been propelled forward by the relentless pursuit of scientific inquiry.

SECTION 1.3

THE ROLE OF NEUROPLASTICITY IN AUDITORY PROCESSING

One of the most remarkable aspects of the auditory system is its capacity for adaptation and change, a phenomenon known as neuroplasticity. Throughout our lives, the neural circuits responsible for processing sound remain malleable and responsive to environmental stimuli, allowing us to fine-tune our auditory abilities in response to new challenges and experiences.

Recent research has shed light on the profound implications of neuroplasticity for auditory health and rehabilitation. Studies have demonstrated that targeted auditory training programs can enhance neural processing and improve speech perception in individuals with hearing impairments. Moreover, advances in neuroimaging technology have provided unprecedented insights into the neural mechanisms underlying auditory plasticity, paving the way for innovative therapies and interventions for individuals with hearing disorders.

By unraveling the mysteries of auditory anatomy and function, we gain a deeper appreciation for the remarkable intricacies of the human auditory system. From the timeless wisdom of ancient scholars to the cutting-edge discoveries of modern science, the study of auditory health continues to evolve, offering new insights and possibilities for the preservation and enhancement of one of our most precious senses.

CHAPTER 2

Understanding Hearing Loss

Hearing loss, a pervasive condition affecting millions worldwide, remains a critical aspect of our sensory health often overlooked. With nearly 50 million individuals grappling with hearing impairment in the United States alone, the significance of comprehending its nuances cannot be overstated. Jennie Boss, drawing from her extensive experience in diagnosing and treating individuals with hearing impairments, sheds light on the multifaceted nature of this sensory deficit.

Join us as we navigate through the labyrinth of auditory complexities, uncovering the delicate interplay between the auditory system's intricate components and the diverse factors contributing to its dysfunction.

SECTION 2.1

THE SPECTRUM OF HEARING LOSS

Hearing loss is a pervasive and multifaceted condition that can manifest across a broad spectrum of severity, from mild impairment to profound deafness. It can arise from a diverse array of factors, including genetic predispositions, environmental exposures, and age-related changes in auditory function. Understanding the different types and causes of hearing loss is essential for effective diagnosis, intervention, and management.

Throughout history, the study of hearing loss has been marked by landmark discoveries and paradigm shifts in our understanding of auditory health. From the pioneering work of Antonio Maria Valsalva in the 18th century, who documented cases of hereditary deafness in his medical observations, to the groundbreaking research of Graeme Clark and his colleagues, whose development of the cochlear implant revolutionized the treatment of severe hearing loss, our knowledge of auditory disorders continues to evolve.

SECTION 2.2

GENETIC FACTORS IN HEARING HEALTH

Genetic factors play a significant role in the development of hearing loss, accounting for a substantial proportion of cases across all age groups. Inherited mutations in genes associated with auditory function can disrupt the delicate mechanisms of the inner ear, leading to progressive sensorineural hearing loss. From congenital disorders such as Waardenburg syndrome, to syndromic conditions like Usher syndrome, the genetic landscape of hearing loss is vast and complex.

Advances in molecular genetics and genomic sequencing have facilitated the identification of genes implicated in hereditary hearing disorders, enabling clinicians to offer tailored genetic counseling and diagnostic testing to individuals and families at risk. Moreover, ongoing research into the genetic basis of hearing loss holds promise for the development of novel therapies and interventions aimed at preserving auditory function and mitigating the progression of genetic hearing disorders.

SECTION 2.3

ENVIRONMENTAL INFLUENCES ON HEARING HEALTH

In addition to genetic factors, environmental exposures can exert a profound impact on auditory health, contributing to the development of acquired hearing loss. Prolonged exposure to loud noise, occupational hazards, and ototoxic medications are among the leading causes of sensorineural hearing loss in adults. Noise-induced hearing loss, in particular, remains a significant public health concern, affecting individuals across all age groups and occupational sectors.

Historically, efforts to mitigate the adverse effects of noise exposure date back to antiquity, with ancient civilizations employing various strategies to protect their ears from the cacophony of battle, industry, and everyday life. In modern times, the recognition of noise-induced hearing loss as a preventable condition has led to the implementation of occupational health and safety regulations, the development of hearing conservation programs, and public awareness campaigns aimed at promoting safe listening practices.

SECTION 2.4

AGE-RELATED HEARING LOSS: PRESERVING SOUND AMIDST TIME

Age-related hearing loss, also known as presbycusis, is a common and often overlooked consequence of the aging process, affecting a significant proportion of older adults worldwide. Characterized by a gradual decline in auditory sensitivity and speech discrimination, presbycusis can have profound implications for communication, social engagement, and quality of life in older individuals.

Throughout history, the phenomenon of age-related hearing loss has been recognized and documented in medical literature dating back to ancient civilizations. From the writings of Hippocrates and Galen, who described the sensory changes associated with aging, to the seminal research of Raymond Carhart and his colleagues, who elucidated the physiological mechanisms underlying presbycusis, our understanding of age-related hearing loss continues to evolve.

By sorting out the complex interplay of genetic, environmental, and age-related factors that contribute to hearing loss, we gain valuable insights into the diverse manifestations of auditory impairment and the myriad challenges faced by individuals with hearing disorders. Through continued research, education, and advocacy, we can strive to mitigate the burden of hearing loss and promote auditory health for individuals of all ages and walks of life.

CHAPTER 3

NOISE POLLUTION AND ITS IMPACT ON HEARING

SECTION 3.1

THE RISE OF NOISE POLLUTION

Noise pollution has emerged as a pervasive and insidious threat to auditory health, permeating our urban landscapes, industrial environments, and everyday surroundings. Defined as unwanted or harmful sound that disrupts the tranquility of the environment, noise pollution can encompass a wide range of sources, including traffic, construction activities, industrial machinery, and recreational activities.

Throughout history, human societies have grappled with the challenges posed by noise pollution, albeit to varying degrees. Ancient civilizations recognized the adverse effects of excessive noise on health and well-being, employing rudimentary measures such as ear coverings and sound-absorbing materials to mitigate its impact. In modern times, the increase of urbanization, industrialization, and technological advancement has intensified the prevalence of noise pollution, posing a significant threat to auditory health on a global scale.

SECTION 3.2

THE PHYSIOLOGY OF NOISE-INDUCED HEARING LOSS

Noise-induced hearing loss (NIHL) is a common and preventable form of sensorineural hearing loss that results from exposure to excessive levels of noise. Prolonged or repeated exposure to high-intensity sounds can damage the delicate hair cells of the cochlea, leading to irreversible hearing loss and auditory dysfunction.

The physiological mechanisms underlying NIHL have been the subject of extensive research and investigation. Studies have shown that exposure to intense noise triggers a cascade of cellular events within the cochlea, including the generation of reactive oxygen species, inflammation, and apoptosis (cell death) of hair cells and supporting structures. Over time, these pathological changes can culminate in the degeneration of auditory nerve fibers and permanent impairment of hearing function.

SECTION 3.3

OCCUPATIONAL HAZARDS AND HEARING PROTECTION

Occupational noise exposure remains a leading cause of NIHL among workers in various industries, including manufacturing, construction, transportation, and agriculture. Workers who are routinely exposed to high levels of noise are at increased risk of developing hearing loss and other auditory disorders, underscoring the importance of effective hearing conservation programs and workplace safety regulations.

Throughout history, efforts to protect workers from the harmful effects of occupational noise have evolved in tandem with advancements in industrialization and labor rights. From the establishment of early noise control measures in 19th-century factories to the development of modern hearing protection devices and engineering controls, occupational health and safety initiatives have played a pivotal role in mitigating the impact of noise pollution on workers' health and well-being.

SECTION 3.4

PUBLIC HEALTH IMPLICATIONS AND POLICY INTERVENTIONS

The public health implications of noise pollution extend far beyond the realm of auditory health, encompassing a broad spectrum of physical, psychological, and social consequences. Chronic exposure to noise has been linked to a range of adverse health outcomes, including cardiovascular disease, sleep disturbances, cognitive impairment, and stress-related disorders.

Recognizing the multifaceted nature of noise pollution, policymakers and public health authorities have implemented a variety of interventions aimed at reducing environmental noise levels and protecting vulnerable populations. These initiatives encompass a diverse array of strategies, including land use planning, noise abatement technologies, community education programs, and regulatory measures to limit noise emissions from transportation and industrial activities.

By addressing the root causes of noise pollution and implementing evidence-based interventions, we can mitigate its adverse effects on auditory health and promote a more tranquil and harmonious living environment for present and future generations. Through collective action and advocacy, we can strive to safeguard our auditory heritage and preserve the precious gift of sound for all.

CHAPTER 4

Genetic Factors in Hearing Health

In some cases, hearing loss can stem from genetic predispositions or hereditary conditions that compromise the integrity of the auditory system. These genetic abnormalities may affect the development or function of the cochlear hair cells, resulting in impaired auditory processing and transmission.

SECTION 4.1

UNRAVELING THE GENETIC LANDSCAPE OF HEARING LOSS

Genetic factors play a pivotal role in the development and progression of hearing loss, contributing to a significant proportion of cases across diverse populations and age groups. From congenital deafness to late-onset sensorineural impairment, hereditary factors can exert a profound influence on auditory function, shaping the susceptibility and severity of hearing disorders.

Historically, the study of genetic hearing loss has undergone remarkable advances, driven by the pioneering efforts of scientists and researchers around the world. Early investigations into familial deafness in the

19th century laid the groundwork for our understanding of hereditary hearing disorders, revealing patterns of inheritance and familial clustering that hinted at underlying genetic mechanisms.

Subsequent discoveries, such as the identification of the connexin 26 gene (GJB2) as a major contributor to non-syndromic autosomal recessive deafness, have deepened our knowledge of the genetic basis of hearing loss and informed diagnostic and therapeutic approaches.

SECTION 4.2

GENETIC VARIANTS ASSOCIATED WITH HEARING DISORDERS

The genetic landscape of hearing loss is characterized by a diverse array of variants and mutations that affect genes involved in auditory development, function, and maintenance. These genetic alterations can disrupt the delicate mechanisms of the inner ear, impairing the transmission of sound signals from the cochlea to the auditory cortex and leading to sensorineural hearing loss.

Recent advances in genomic sequencing technologies have facilitated the identification of numerous genes implicated in hereditary hearing disorders, offering new insights into the molecular mechanisms underlying auditory dysfunction. Mutations in genes encoding components of the cochlear hair cells, such as MYO7A and USH2A, are associated with syndromic forms of deafness, while variants in genes involved in ion channel function, such as KCNQ4 and SLC26A4, are linked to non-syndromic forms of hearing loss.

The elucidation of these genetic pathways and molecular pathways has paved the way for personalized approaches to diagnosis, prognosis, and treatment of hereditary hearing disorders. Genetic testing and counseling have become integral components of clinical care for individuals with suspected genetic hearing loss, enabling healthcare providers to tailor interventions and support services to meet the unique needs of patients and their families.

SECTION 4.3

EMERGING THERAPEUTIC STRATEGIES FOR GENETIC HEARING LOSS

The advent of precision medicine and gene therapy holds promise for the treatment and management of genetic hearing loss, offering new avenues for targeted interventions and therapeutic interventions. Experimental approaches, such as gene editing technologies and viral vectors, have shown potential for correcting genetic defects and restoring auditory function in preclinical models of hereditary deafness.

In recent years, landmark achievements in gene therapy have propelled the field of genetic hearing loss research forward, with clinical trials demonstrating the feasibility and safety of gene-based interventions for selected forms of inherited deafness. The development of innovative delivery methods and gene editing tools, such as CRISPR-Cas9, heralds a new era of personalized medicine for individuals with genetic hearing disorders, offering hope for improved outcomes and quality of life.

By extrication the intricate genetic pathways that underlie hearing loss and leveraging cutting-edge technologies to develop targeted therapies, we can pave the way for a future where genetic hearing disorders are treated with precision and compassion. Through collaborative research efforts and interdisciplinary collaboration, we can harness the power of genetics to unlock new possibilities for auditory health and well-being for generations to come.

CHAPTER 5

AGE-RELATED HEARING LOSS: PRESERVING SOUND AMIDST TIME

SECTION 5.1

THE PHENOMENON OF AGE-RELATED HEARING LOSS

Age-related hearing loss, also known as presbycusis, is a common and often overlooked consequence of the aging process, affecting a significant proportion of older adults worldwide. Characterized by a gradual decline in auditory sensitivity and speech discrimination, presbycusis can have profound implications for communication, social engagement, and quality of life in older individuals.

Historically, the phenomenon of age-related hearing loss has been recognized and documented in medical literature dating back centuries. Ancient texts, including the writings of Hippocrates and Galen, described the sensory changes associated with aging, noting the gradual decline in auditory acuity and the prevalence of hearing impairment among elderly populations. Throughout the ages, scholars and physicians have sought to unravel the mysteries of presbycusis, exploring its underlying mechanisms and developing strategies for prevention and management.

SECTION 5.2

THE PHYSIOLOGY OF AGE-RELATED HEARING LOSS

The physiological mechanisms underlying age-related hearing loss are multifaceted and complex, reflecting a combination of genetic predispositions, environmental exposures, and cumulative damage to the auditory system over time. As individuals age, the delicate structures of the inner ear, including the cochlea and auditory nerve fibers, undergo degenerative changes that compromise their function and integrity.

Studies have shown that age-related changes in the cochlea, such as loss of sensory hair cells, thinning of the stria vascularis, and fibrosis of the basilar membrane, contribute to the progressive decline in auditory sensitivity and frequency resolution associated with presbycusis. Moreover, alterations in central auditory processing pathways and synaptic connectivity within the brain can further exacerbate age-related auditory deficits, impairing speech perception and sound localization in older adults.

SECTION 5.3

RISK FACTORS AND PROTECTIVE FACTORS FOR AGE-RELATED HEARING LOSS

While age is the primary risk factor for presbycusis, numerous additional factors can influence the onset and progression of age-related hearing loss. Chronic exposure to noise, ototoxic medications, and environmental toxins can accelerate the degenerative processes in the inner ear, exacerbating age-related auditory dysfunction. Moreover, systemic conditions such as diabetes, hypertension, and cardiovascular disease have been implicated in the pathogenesis of presbycusis, underscoring the complex interplay between auditory health and overall wellness.

Conversely, certain lifestyle factors and protective behaviors may help mitigate the risk of age-related hearing loss and preserve auditory function in older individuals. Maintaining a healthy diet rich in antioxidants and essential nutrients, engaging in regular physical activity, and avoiding exposure to excessive noise can promote optimal auditory health and reduce the likelihood of age-related auditory decline.

Moreover, the use of hearing protection devices and regular monitoring of hearing status through audiometric screenings can facilitate early detection and intervention for age-related hearing loss.

SECTION 5.4

STRATEGIES FOR PREVENTION AND MANAGEMENT

Preventing age-related hearing loss and mitigating its impact requires a comprehensive and multifaceted approach that addresses both individual and societal factors. Public health initiatives aimed at promoting awareness of age-related hearing loss, fostering healthy aging practices, and advocating for accessible hearing healthcare services can help reduce the burden of presbycusis and improve the quality of life for older adults.

Clinical interventions for age-related hearing loss may include hearing aids, assistive listening devices, and auditory rehabilitation programs designed to enhance speech perception and auditory communication in older individuals. Moreover, emerging technologies such as cochlear implants and auditory brainstem implants offer promising options for individuals with severe or profound age-related hearing loss who may benefit from surgical intervention.

By embracing a holistic approach to age-related hearing loss, grounded in scientific evidence and compassionate care, we can empower older adults to maintain their auditory independence, engage fully in social and cognitive activities, and enjoy a life enriched by the beauty of sound. Through continued research, advocacy, and innovation, we can ensure that the golden years are truly golden, filled with the joy of music, conversation, and connection for generations to come.

CHAPTER 6

Occupational Hazards and Hearing Protection

Mitigating exposure to excessively loud environments through the consistent use of hearing protection devices, such as earplugs or earmuffs, serves as a primary preventive measure against noise-induced sensorineural hearing loss.

SECTION 6.1

The Historical Context of Occupational Noise Exposure

Stakeholders have recognized exposure to occupational noise as a significant occupational hazard throughout history. It results in workers in various industries facing heightened risk of hearing loss and auditory impairment. From the clangor of early industrial machinery to the roar of modern manufacturing processes, noise has long been a ubiquitous presence in the workplace, posing a threat to the auditory health and well-being of workers around the world.

In the past, we often overlooked or underestimated the detrimental effects of occupational noise exposure. The employers and policymakers failed to recognize the long-term consequences of prolonged exposure to high-intensity sound. It was not until the early 20th century that pioneering researchers and advocates began to raise awareness of the link between occupational noise and hearing loss. They began advocating for legislative measures and workplace reforms to protect workers from the harmful effects of noise pollution.

SECTION 6.2

THE PHYSIOLOGY OF NOISE-INDUCED HEARING LOSS

Noise-induced hearing loss (NIHL) is a common and preventable form of sensorineural hearing loss that results from exposure to excessive levels of noise in the workplace. Prolonged or repeated exposure to high-intensity sounds can damage the delicate hair cells of the cochlea, leading to irreversible hearing loss and auditory dysfunction.

The physiological mechanisms underlying NIHL are complex and multifaceted, involving a cascade of cellular events within the cochlea in response to intense noise exposure. Studies have shown that exposure to loud noise triggers the generation of reactive oxygen species, inflammation, and cellular apoptosis (programmed cell death) in the cochlear hair cells and supporting structures. Over time, these pathological changes can culminate in the degeneration of auditory nerve fibers and permanent impairment of hearing function.

SECTION 6.3

OCCUPATIONAL SECTORS AT RISK

Workers in a variety of industries are at increased risk of occupational noise exposure and subsequent hearing loss. Manufacturing, construction, mining, transportation, agriculture, and entertainment are among the sectors with the highest prevalence of hazardous noise levels, placing employees at heightened risk of NIHL and other auditory disorders.

Throughout history, efforts to mitigate the adverse effects of occupational noise exposure have evolved in tandem with advancements in industrialization and labor rights. From the enactment of early noise control measures in 19th-century factories to the development of modern hearing conservation programs and occupational health and safety regulations, employers and policymakers have sought to protect workers from the harmful effects of noise pollution.

SECTION 6.4

HEARING PROTECTION STRATEGIES AND INTERVENTIONS

Hearing protection strategies play a crucial role in mitigating the risk of occupational noise-induced hearing loss and promoting auditory health in the workplace. Personal protective equipment, such as earplugs and earmuffs, serves as the frontline defense against hazardous noise exposure, providing a physical barrier to attenuate sound levels and safeguard the delicate structures of the inner ear.

In addition to personal protective equipment, engineering controls and administrative measures can help reduce noise levels and minimize exposure in noisy work environments. Noise control technologies, such as sound insulation, vibration damping, and machinery enclosures, can mitigate the propagation of noise and limit the spread of hazardous sound emissions. Moreover, workplace policies and education programs aimed at promoting safe listening practices and raising awareness of the importance of hearing conservation can empower employees to take proactive steps to protect their auditory health.

By embracing a comprehensive approach to hearing protection and occupational safety, employers, policymakers, and healthcare professionals can create healthier and more sustainable work environments that prioritize the well-being and dignity of workers. Through collaborative efforts and evidence-based interventions, we can strive to mitigate the burden of occupational noise-induced hearing loss and ensure that every worker has the opportunity to thrive in a safe and supportive workplace.

CHAPTER 7

LIFESTYLE CHOICES FOR HEARING WELLNESS

Adopting a healthy lifestyle characterized by balanced nutrition, regular exercise, and avoidance of ototoxic substances can promote overall well-being and mitigate the risk factors associated with sensorineural hearing loss. Individuals are encouraged to prioritize self-care practices that prioritize auditory health and resilience.

SECTION 7.1

THE IMPACT OF LIFESTYLE ON AUDITORY HEALTH

Lifestyle choices play a significant role in determining the long-term health and well-being of our auditory system. From dietary habits and physical activity to recreational activities and environmental exposures, the choices we make in our daily lives can profoundly influence our susceptibility to hearing loss and auditory impairment.

Throughout history, societies have recognized the importance of healthy living practices in promoting overall wellness, including auditory health. Ancient civilizations such as the Greeks and Romans valued moderation and balance in diet and exercise. They often acknowledged the interconnectedness of physical and sensory well-being.

Over time, advances in scientific research and medical knowledge have deepened our understanding of the complex relationship between lifestyle factors and auditory function. Thus, informing preventive strategies and intervention approaches for hearing wellness.

SECTION 7.2

DIET AND NUTRITION FOR AUDITORY HEALTH

Diet and nutrition play a crucial role in supporting the delicate structures of the inner ear and preserving auditory function throughout life. Essential nutrients such as vitamins A, C, and E, as well as minerals like magnesium and zinc, contribute to the maintenance of healthy cochlear hair cells and the integrity of auditory nerve fibers.

Historically, traditional diets rich in fruits, vegetables, whole grains, and lean proteins have been associated with improved auditory health and reduced risk of hearing loss. Ancient cultures such as the Mediterranean and Japanese civilizations embraced plant-based diets and seafood-rich cuisines, recognizing the potential benefits of nutrient-dense foods in promoting sensory acuity and longevity.

Contemporary research has underscored the importance of a balanced and diverse diet in supporting auditory wellness. Studies have shown that antioxidants, found abundantly in fruits and vegetables, can help protect against oxidative stress and cellular damage in the cochlea, while omega-3 fatty acids, abundant in fish and nuts, may contribute to the preservation of auditory function and prevention of age-related hearing loss.

SECTION 7.3

PHYSICAL ACTIVITY AND CARDIOVASCULAR HEALTH

Regular physical activity and cardiovascular fitness are integral components of a healthy lifestyle and can have profound implications for auditory health. Maintaining optimal cardiovascular function supports efficient blood flow to the cochlea and auditory structures, ensuring adequate oxygenation and nutrient delivery to support cellular metabolism and repair processes.

Throughout history, physical activity has been revered as a cornerstone of well-being, with ancient civilizations such as the Egyptians and Chinese embracing exercise as a means of promoting vitality and longevity. From the martial arts of Asia to the Olympic games of ancient Greece, cultures around the world have celebrated the transformative power of movement and athleticism in shaping mind, body, and spirit.

Contemporary research has highlighted the cardiovascular benefits of regular exercise in preserving auditory function and reducing the risk of age-related hearing loss. Studies have shown that individuals who engage in moderate-to-vigorous physical activity experience lower rates of hearing impairment and auditory decline compared to sedentary counterparts, underscoring the importance of incorporating regular exercise into daily routines for optimal auditory wellness.

SECTION 7.4

ENVIRONMENTAL EXPOSURES AND HEALTHY HABITS

In addition to diet and exercise, environmental exposures and lifestyle habits can impact auditory health and contribute to the risk of hearing loss and auditory dysfunction. Avoiding exposure to excessive noise, limiting use of ototoxic medications, and refraining from smoking and excessive alcohol consumption are important strategies for preserving auditory function and reducing the likelihood of hearing impairment.

History recorded that societies have recognized the adverse effects of environmental toxins and unhealthy behaviors on sensory health, implementing cultural norms and social customs to promote responsible living practices. Ancient cultures such as the Native Americans and Aboriginal Australians revered the natural world and embraced harmonious relationships with their environment, emphasizing stewardship and sustainability in daily life.

Contemporary public health initiatives and educational campaigns promote awareness of the impact of environmental exposures and lifestyle choices on auditory health. From workplace safety regulations to community outreach programs, efforts to raise awareness of noise-induced hearing loss, promote hearing conservation, and advocate for healthy living habits aim to empower individuals and communities to prioritize auditory wellness and preserve the precious gift of hearing for generations to come.

By embracing a holistic approach to hearing wellness and adopting healthy lifestyle practices, individuals can optimize their auditory health and enhance their quality of life. Through education, advocacy, and community engagement, we can foster a culture of prevention and empowerment, where every individual has the opportunity to thrive and experience the richness of sound in all its beauty and diversity.

CHAPTER 8

THE ROLE OF DIET AND NUTRITION IN AUDITORY HEALTH

SECTION 8.1

UNDERSTANDING THE RELATIONSHIP BETWEEN DIET AND AUDITORY WELLNESS

Diet and nutrition play a crucial role in maintaining optimal auditory health and preventing the onset of hearing loss and auditory disorders. The nutrients we consume through our diet provide essential building blocks for the intricate structures of the inner ear, support cellular metabolism and repair processes, and help protect against oxidative stress and inflammation, which can contribute to auditory dysfunction.

Throughout history, cultures around the world have recognized the importance of dietary practices in promoting overall well-being, including sensory health. Ancient civilizations such as the Egyptians, Greeks, and Chinese emphasized the therapeutic properties of certain foods and herbs in treating ailments and promoting longevity. Over time, scientific research and medical advancements have deepened our understanding of the intricate interplay between diet, nutrition, and auditory function. This makes it easier to adopt timely preventive strategies and intervention approaches for hearing wellness.

SECTION 8.2

ESSENTIAL NUTRIENTS FOR AUDITORY HEALTH

A balanced and diverse diet rich in essential nutrients is critical for supporting the delicate structures of the inner ear and preserving auditory function throughout life. Key nutrients that play a pivotal role in auditory health include vitamins A, C, and E, as well as minerals such as magnesium, zinc, and selenium.

Vitamin A, found in abundance in colorful fruits and vegetables, is essential for maintaining the health of the auditory nerve fibers and supporting the transmission of sound signals to the brain. Vitamin C, present in citrus fruits, strawberries, and bell peppers, acts as a powerful antioxidant, protecting against oxidative stress and cellular damage in the cochlea. Vitamin E, found in nuts, seeds, and leafy greens, helps maintain the integrity of the cochlear hair cells and supports auditory function.

Minerals such as magnesium, zinc, and selenium play critical roles in regulating cellular metabolism and protecting against age-related oxidative damage in the auditory system. Magnesium, abundant in green leafy vegetables, whole grains, and nuts, helps maintain the elasticity of the cochlear blood vessels and supports efficient nutrient delivery to the inner ear.

Others include Zinc found in shellfish, meat, and legumes, which plays a key role in the synthesis of proteins and enzymes involved in auditory neurotransmission.

Selenium, present in seafood, Brazil nuts, and eggs, acts as a cofactor for antioxidant enzymes, protecting against oxidative stress and cellular damage in the cochlea.

SECTION 8.3

DIETARY PATTERNS AND AUDITORY WELLNESS

In addition to individual nutrients, dietary patterns and overall dietary quality also play a significant role in auditory health. Diets rich in fruits, vegetables, whole grains, lean proteins, and healthy fats have been associated with improved auditory function and reduced risk of hearing loss and auditory disorders.

In the past, traditional dietary patterns such as the Mediterranean diet and the DASH (Dietary Approaches to Stop Hypertension) diet have been lauded for their potential benefits in promoting sensory acuity and longevity. These dietary patterns emphasize consumption of plant-based foods, seafood, nuts, and olive oil, while limiting intake of processed foods, red meat, and sugary beverages.

Contemporary research supports the role of dietary patterns in preserving auditory function and reducing the risk of age-related hearing loss. Studies have shown that individuals who adhere to healthy dietary patterns, such as the Mediterranean diet or the Dietary Approaches to Stop Hypertension (DASH) diet, experience lower rates of hearing impairment and auditory decline compared to those with less optimal dietary habits.

SECTION 8.4

PRACTICAL RECOMMENDATIONS FOR AUDITORY WELLNESS

Incorporating nutrient-rich foods into your daily diet is an essential step in promoting auditory health and preserving the precious gift of hearing. Aim to consume a diverse array of fruits, vegetables, whole grains, lean proteins, and healthy fats to ensure adequate intake of essential nutrients for auditory function.

Choose colorful fruits and vegetables such as berries, citrus fruits, spinach, and sweet potatoes, which are rich in vitamins A and C, as well as antioxidants that protect against oxidative stress and cellular damage in the cochlea. Incorporate sources of omega-3 fatty acids such as fatty fish (salmon, mackerel, sardines), flaxseeds, and walnuts into your diet to support cardiovascular health and promote optimal blood flow to the inner ear.

Limit consumption of processed foods, sugary beverages, and foods high in saturated and trans fats, which can contribute to inflammation and oxidative stress in the body and impair auditory function. Be mindful of your salt intake and opt for low-sodium options to help maintain healthy blood pressure levels and reduce the risk of cochlear damage associated with hypertension.

By adopting a balanced and nutrient-rich diet, you can support the health and vitality of your auditory system and enjoy the beauty of sound in all its richness and diversity. Through informed dietary choices and a commitment to holistic wellness, you can preserve the precious gift of hearing and enhance your quality of life for years to come.

CHAPTER 9

THE IMPACT OF ENVIRONMENTAL FACTORS ON AUDITORY HEALTH

SECTION 9.1

UNDERSTANDING ENVIRONMENTAL INFLUENCES ON HEARING

Environmental factors play a significant role in shaping auditory health and contributing to the risk of hearing loss and auditory disorders. From exposure to loud noise and ototoxic chemicals to air pollution and climate change, the environment in which we live can exert profound effects on the delicate structures of the inner ear and the function of the auditory system.

Historically, societies have grappled with the challenges posed by environmental pollutants and hazards to sensory health, recognizing the importance of preserving the natural world and safeguarding human health from harmful exposures.

Ancient civilizations such as the Romans and Greeks valued the therapeutic properties of natural environments and advocated for the preservation of clean air and water sources as essential elements of well-being. Over time, industrialization, urbanization, and technological advancements have introduced new environmental stressors and pollutants that pose threats to auditory wellness.

SECTION 9.2

NOISE POLLUTION: A GLOBAL CHALLENGE

Noise pollution is one of the most pervasive environmental threats to auditory health, affecting millions of individuals worldwide and contributing to the burden of hearing loss and auditory dysfunction. Defined as unwanted or harmful sound that disrupts the tranquility of the environment, noise pollution can emanate from a variety of sources, including traffic, industrial activities, construction sites, and recreational pursuits.

Throughout history, societies have contended with the adverse effects of noise pollution on human health and well-being, recognizing the deleterious impact of excessive noise on auditory function and quality of life. Ancient civilizations employed various strategies to mitigate noise pollution, including zoning regulations, sound barriers, and restrictions on noisy activities in residential areas.

In modern times, the proliferation of urbanization, transportation networks, and industrial facilities has intensified the prevalence of noise pollution, prompting calls for stricter regulations and public awareness campaigns to address this growing public health concern.

SECTION 9.3

OTOTOXIC CHEMICALS AND ENVIRONMENTAL TOXINS

In addition to noise pollution, exposure to ototoxic chemicals and environmental toxins can pose significant risks to auditory health and contribute to the development of hearing loss and auditory disorders. Ototoxic substances, such as certain medications, industrial chemicals, and heavy metals, have the potential to damage the delicate structures of the inner ear and impair auditory function.

Societies have recognized the dangers posed by ototoxic chemicals and environmental toxins to sensory health, implementing regulations and guidelines to minimize exposure and mitigate risks.

Ancient cultures such as the Egyptians and Greeks documented the toxic effects of certain substances on sensory function and advocated for caution in their use.

In modern times, advances in industrialization and chemical manufacturing have introduced new ototoxic hazards, prompting efforts to identify and regulate potentially harmful substances in the environment.

SECTION 9.4

CLIMATE CHANGE AND AUDITORY WELLNESS

Climate change represents a growing threat to auditory health, with rising temperatures, extreme weather events, and environmental disruptions posing risks to the auditory system and exacerbating existing vulnerabilities. Changes in climate patterns can impact environmental noise levels, air quality, and exposure to environmental toxins, potentially leading to adverse effects on auditory function and well-being.

Most societies have grappled with the complex interplay between climate change and human health, recognizing the interconnectedness of environmental sustainability and public health. Ancient cultures such as the Mayans and Incas observed changes in weather patterns and environmental conditions and adapted their lifestyles and practices to mitigate risks and ensure survival.

In modern times, the recognition of climate change as a global challenge has prompted efforts to reduce greenhouse gas emissions, promote renewable energy sources, and mitigate the impacts of environmental degradation on human health.

By understanding the multifaceted nature of environmental influences on auditory health and adopting proactive measures to mitigate risks and promote resilience, we can safeguard the precious gift of hearing for generations to come. Through collaborative efforts and informed decision-making, we can foster a healthier and more sustainable environment that supports the well-being and vitality of all.

CHAPTER 10

INNOVATIONS IN HEARING TECHNOLOGY AND REHABILITATION

SECTION 10.1

THE EVOLUTION OF HEARING TECHNOLOGY

The field of hearing technology has undergone remarkable advancements throughout history, revolutionizing the diagnosis, treatment, and rehabilitation of auditory disorders. From the invention of the first hearing aids to the development of sophisticated cochlear implant systems, innovations in hearing technology have transformed the lives of millions of individuals with hearing loss around the world.

The earliest attempts to address hearing impairment date back centuries, with rudimentary hearing aids made from natural materials such as animal horns, shells, and wood. In the 17th and 18th centuries, the invention of mechanical ear trumpets and speaking tubes provided crude amplification for individuals with hearing loss, marking the beginnings of modern hearing aid technology.

The 20th century witnessed dramatic advances in hearing technology, fueled by scientific discoveries, technological innovation, and the growing demand for effective solutions to hearing impairment. From the development of vacuum tube hearing aids in the early 1900s, to the introduction of transistor-based devices in the mid-20th century, each successive generation of hearing technology brought improvements in size, performance, and functionality.

SECTION 10.2

CONTEMPORARY HEARING AID TECHNOLOGY

Contemporary hearing aids represent the pinnacle of technological innovation, offering a wide range of features and capabilities to address the diverse needs of individuals with hearing loss. Modern hearing aids utilize digital signal processing algorithms, wireless connectivity, and adaptive processing techniques to deliver personalized amplification and enhance speech understanding in various listening environments.

In recent years, the miniaturization of components and advances in microelectronics has enabled the development of discreet and cosmetically appealing hearing aids that are virtually invisible when worn. Bluetooth connectivity and smartphone compatibility allow users to stream audio directly to their hearing aids from smartphones, TVs, and other electronic devices, enhancing accessibility and convenience.

Furthermore, adaptive processing algorithms and artificial intelligence technologies enable hearing aids to adjust automatically settings in real time based on the acoustic environment, optimizing speech intelligibility and reducing background noise. Telehealth platforms and remote programming capabilities allow audiologists to remotely adjust and fine-tune hearing aids, providing greater flexibility and convenience for users.

SECTION 10.3

COCHLEAR IMPLANTS: RESTORING AUDITORY FUNCTION

Cochlear implants represent a groundbreaking innovation in auditory rehabilitation, offering a life-changing solution for individuals with severe to profound sensorineural hearing loss. Unlike traditional hearing aids, which amplify sound for residual hearing, cochlear implants bypass damaged hair cells in the cochlea and directly stimulate the auditory nerve, restoring the perception of sound.

The development of the first cochlear implant by Professor Graeme Clark and his team in the 1970s marked a major milestone in the treatment of profound deafness, paving the way for subsequent generations of cochlear implant technology. Today, cochlear implants consist of an external speech processor and internal electrode array. Surgically, we implant these into the cochlea, enabling individuals with severe hearing loss to perceive speech and environmental sounds.

Advancements in cochlear implant technology have led to improvements in speech understanding, sound quality, and durability, expanding the candidacy criteria and improving outcomes for recipients of all ages.

Bilateral cochlear implantation, simultaneous auditory processing strategies, and electrodes array design optimization have further enhanced the efficacy and usability of cochlear implants, enabling individuals with severe to profound hearing loss to communicate effectively and participate fully in everyday life.

SECTION 10.4

EMERGING TRENDS AND FUTURE DIRECTIONS

The future of hearing technology holds promise for continued innovation and advancement, driven by ongoing research, technological breakthroughs, and the evolving needs of individuals with hearing loss. Emerging trends such as bone conduction implants, hybrid cochlear implants, and regenerative medicine approaches offer new avenues for restoring auditory function and improving outcomes for individuals with sensorineural hearing loss.

Moreover, advancements in telehealth, artificial intelligence, and machine learning hold potential for enhancing diagnostic accuracy, personalized treatment planning, and rehabilitation outcomes for individuals with hearing loss. Virtual reality simulations, immersive auditory training programs, and interactive listening exercises provide innovative tools for auditory rehabilitation and cognitive training, enabling individuals to optimize their auditory skills and adapt to challenging listening environments.

By embracing a spirit of innovation, collaboration, and compassion, we can harness the power of technology to transform the lives of individuals with hearing loss and empower them to engage fully in the world of sound. Through continued research, advocacy, and investment in hearing healthcare, we can ensure that individuals of all ages and backgrounds have access to the life-changing benefits of cutting-edge hearing technology and rehabilitation services.

CHAPTER 11

THE IMPORTANCE OF EARLY INTERVENTION IN HEARING HEALTH

SECTION 11.1

THE SIGNIFICANCE OF EARLY DETECTION

Early intervention plays a crucial role in mitigating the impact of hearing loss and promoting optimal auditory health outcomes. Timely identification and management of hearing impairment in infants, children, and adults can facilitate language development, academic achievement, and social-emotional well-being, laying the foundation for a lifetime of communication and learning.

Healthcare professionals, educators, and policymakers around the world have recognized the importance of early detection of hearing loss. In the late 19th and early 20th centuries, pioneering researchers such as Dr. Arnold Gesell and Dr. William House conducted groundbreaking studies on early childhood development and auditory function, highlighting the critical period for language acquisition and the importance of early intervention in addressing hearing loss.

SECTION 11.2

SCREENING AND DIAGNOSTIC TOOLS

Effective early intervention relies on the availability of screening and diagnostic tools that enable healthcare providers to identify hearing loss accurately and efficiently. Newborn hearing screening programs, implemented in many countries around the world, use objective measures such as otoacoustic emissions (OAE) and auditory brainstem response (ABR) testing to assess auditory function shortly after birth, allowing for early detection of congenital hearing loss.

In addition to newborn screening, routine hearing evaluations and audiometric assessments play a crucial role in monitoring auditory health and identifying hearing loss in children and adults. Pure-tone audiometry, speech audiometry, tympanometry, and acoustic emittance testing are among the diagnostic tools used by audiologists to evaluate hearing sensitivity, speech perception, middle ear function, and auditory processing abilities.

Furthermore, advances in technology have led to the development of portable, smartphone-based hearing screening applications and tele audiology platforms that enable remote assessment and monitoring of auditory function, expanding access to early intervention services in underserved communities and remote regions.

SECTION 11.3

INTERVENTION STRATEGIES FOR CHILDREN

Early intervention services for children with hearing loss encompass a continuum of care that includes amplification, auditory habilitation, speech-language therapy, educational support, and family-centered intervention. Hearing aids and cochlear implants are among the most common amplification options for children with sensorineural hearing loss, providing access to auditory information and facilitating speech and language development.

Speech-language therapy and auditory-verbal therapy play a central role in promoting auditory skill development and communication competence in children with hearing loss. These interventions focus on maximizing auditory potential, improving speech intelligibility, and fostering age-appropriate language acquisition through structured activities, play-based learning, and family involvement.

Educational accommodations and support services, such as classroom amplification systems, FM systems, and assistive listening devices, help ensure that children with hearing loss have equal access to educational opportunities and academic success. Early childhood intervention programs, preschool programs for children with hearing loss, and mainstream educational settings with appropriate support services provide opportunities for socialization, peer interaction, and academic achievement.

SECTION 11.4

EMPOWERING ADULTS THROUGH EARLY INTERVENTION

Early intervention is equally important

for adults with hearing loss, as it can prevent the negative consequences associated with untreated hearing impairment and improve overall quality of life. Adults who experience changes in their hearing should seek prompt evaluation by an audiologist to determine the extent and nature of their hearing loss and explore appropriate treatment options.

Hearing aids, assistive listening devices, and communication strategies are among the interventions available to adults with hearing loss, enabling them to overcome communication barriers and participate fully in social, occupational, and recreational activities. Counseling and support services, including auditory rehabilitation programs and peer support groups, help individuals adjust to life with hearing loss and develop coping strategies for managing everyday challenges.

Moreover, addressing hearing loss early can reduce the risk of cognitive decline, social isolation, depression, and other negative outcomes associated with untreated hearing impairment. By empowering individuals to take proactive steps to address their hearing health needs, early intervention can enhance overall well-being and promote active engagement in all aspects of life.

Through concerted efforts to promote awareness, access, and affordability of early intervention services, we can ensure that individuals of all ages and backgrounds have the opportunity to benefit from timely detection and management of hearing loss.

By prioritizing early intervention in hearing health, we can empower individuals to unlock their full potential and thrive in a world enriched by the beauty of sound.

CHAPTER 12

CULTIVATING A CULTURE OF HEARING WELLNESS

SECTION 12.1

RECOGNIZING THE IMPORTANCE OF HEARING WELLNESS

Hearing wellness encompasses more than just the absence of hearing loss; it reflects a holistic approach to auditory health that emphasizes prevention, early detection, intervention, and advocacy. Cultivating a culture of hearing wellness involves fostering awareness, promoting education, and advocating for policies and practices that prioritize auditory health and well-being for individuals and communities.

Throughout history, societies have recognized the intrinsic value of hearing as a fundamental aspect of human communication, connection, and engagement with the world. Ancient cultures such as the Greeks and Egyptians revered the power of speech and sound, celebrating the beauty of music, poetry, and oral traditions in their daily lives. Over time, advances in science, technology, and medicine have deepened our understanding of the complexities of auditory function and the importance of preserving hearing for generations to come.

SECTION 12.2

PROMOTING AWARENESS AND EDUCATION

Promoting awareness and education about hearing health is essential for fostering a culture of hearing wellness and empowering individuals to take proactive steps to protect their auditory health. Public awareness campaigns, educational initiatives, and community outreach programs play a crucial role in raising awareness of the importance of hearing conservation, promoting healthy listening habits, and dispelling myths and misconceptions about hearing loss.

According to history, organizations such as the American Speech-Language-Hearing Association (ASHA), the World Health Organization (WHO), and the Hearing Loss

Association of America (HLAA) have been at the forefront of advocacy and education efforts to promote hearing wellness and prevent hearing loss.

Through public service announcements, informational resources, and grassroots advocacy campaigns, these organizations strive to empower individuals with knowledge and resources to make informed decisions about their auditory health.

SECTION 12.3

ADVOCATING FOR ACCESSIBLE HEARING HEALTHCARE

Advocating for accessible hearing healthcare services is essential for ensuring that individuals of all ages and backgrounds have access to timely and affordable hearing screening, diagnosis, intervention, and rehabilitation services. Advocacy efforts aimed at reducing barriers to care, improving insurance coverage, and increasing funding for hearing healthcare programs can help expand access to essential services and improve outcomes for individuals with hearing loss.

Advocacy organizations and professional associations have played a vital role in advocating for policy changes and legislative reforms to enhance access to hearing healthcare services. The passage of laws such as the Americans with Disabilities Act (ADA) in the United States and the implementation of universal newborn hearing screening programs in many countries reflect the growing recognition of the importance of accessible and inclusive hearing healthcare for individuals with hearing loss.

SECTION 12.4

FOSTERING SUPPORTIVE ENVIRONMENTS AND COMMUNITIES

Fostering supportive environments and communities that value and prioritize hearing wellness is essential for creating a culture that embraces diversity, inclusivity, and accessibility for individuals with hearing loss. Communities that promote positive attitudes toward hearing health, provide social support networks, and offer resources for communication access can empower individuals with hearing loss to live full and meaningful lives.

According to history, cultural traditions, social customs, and community norms have played a significant role in shaping attitudes toward hearing health and inclusion of individuals with hearing loss in society. From the establishment of deaf schools and sign language communities to the integration of captioning and assistive listening technologies in public spaces, communities around the world have demonstrated a commitment to fostering environments that support the needs of individuals with hearing loss.

By cultivating a culture of hearing wellness that values prevention, early intervention, accessibility, and inclusivity, we can create a world where individuals of all ages and backgrounds can fully participate in the rich tapestry of human communication and experience the joy of sound in all its beauty and diversity. Through collective efforts and shared commitment to auditory health, we can ensure that hearing wellness remains a priority for generations to come.

CONCLUSION

The journey through the exploration of hearing wellness has revealed the intricate interplay between historical context, scientific advancement, and societal attitudes toward auditory health. From ancient civilizations that revered the power of speech and sound to modern societies grappling with the complexities of hearing loss and auditory impairment, the quest for auditory wellness has been shaped by a myriad of factors, including culture, technology, and public policy.

Throughout history, individuals with hearing loss have faced unique challenges and barriers to participation in everyday life, from communication difficulties and social isolation to limited access to healthcare services and educational opportunities. The recognition of hearing loss as a public health issue has prompted concerted efforts to promote awareness, expand access to care, and advocate for policies and practices that prioritize auditory health and well-being for all.

In recent decades, technological advancements have revolutionized the landscape of hearing healthcare, offering innovative solutions and interventions to address the diverse needs of individuals with hearing loss. From the development of digital hearing aids and cochlear implants to the emergence of tele audiology platforms and assistive listening devices, technology has opened new pathways for diagnosis, treatment, and rehabilitation, empowering individuals to overcome barriers and achieve optimal auditory function.

However, despite significant progress in the field of hearing technology, challenges remain in addressing the unique needs of individuals with hearing loss, including those with special needs and complex communication disorders. The diversity of hearing loss experiences and the intersectionality of factors such as age, language, culture, and socioeconomic status underscore the need for personalized, patient-centered approaches to care that recognize and respect the individuality of each person.

As we look to the future, the quest for auditory wellness must encompass a commitment to equity, inclusion, and accessibility for individuals with hearing loss, including those with special needs and communication challenges. Technological innovation holds tremendous promise for addressing these needs, with emerging technologies such as artificial intelligence, machine learning, and wearable devices offering new opportunities for personalized intervention and support.

By harnessing the power of technology, embracing a culture of compassion and inclusivity, and advocating for policies that prioritize auditory health and well-being, we can create a world where individuals of all ages and backgrounds can thrive in a society that values and respects the richness of human communication and the beauty of sound. Through collaborative efforts and shared commitment to hearing wellness, we can build a brighter future where every voice is heard, and every ear is valued.